DANIEL MPIANA NKONGOLO

Smoking In Pregnant Women

DANIEL MPIANA NKONGOLO

Smoking In Pregnant Women

Smoking In Kinshasa University Clinics And Ngaba Mother And Child Hospital Center

ScienciaScripts

Imprint

Cover image: www.ingimage.com

This book is a translation from the original published under ISBN 978-620-6-73117-7.

Publisher:
Sciencia Scripts
is a trademark of
Dodo Books Indian Ocean Ltd. and OmniScriptum S.R.L publishing group

120 High Road, East Finchley, London, N2 9ED, United Kingdom
Str. Armeneasca 28/1, office 1, Chisinau MD-2012, Republic of Moldova, Europe
Managing Directors: Ieva Konstantinova, Victoria Ursu
info@omniscriptum.com

Printed at: see last page
ISBN: 978-620-8-62538-2

TABLE OF CONTENTS

EPIGRAPH

Sometimes it's easier said than done, and no matter how motivated you , it's hard to put out your cigarette butt just once.

FIGARO

DEDICATION

To my very dear father Florent MPIANA of happy memory, for all his sacrifices, love, tenderness, rigour, support and prayers.

To my dearest mother, Yvette Claire TSHILANDA, for all that you have been and are to me; you gave everything you could for my excellence.

To my sister Merveille MPIANA, of happy memory, who showed her true love for me, her support, attention and many pieces of advice and remarks shaped me, I keep your precious image, because you are a perpetual source of motivation.

ACKNOWLEDGEMENTS

We would like to express our gratitude to the members of the Management Committee and the dean's authorities of the Faculty Medicine in general, as well as the teaching staff, for ensuring our continuing education throughout our academic career at the UNIVESRITE DE KINSHASA, our alma mater.

We would like to express our gratitude to our promoter, Professor Dr. Damien MBANZULU PITA, for the sacrifices he made and the support he provided for the preparation of this work, despite his many commitments.

We would like to thank Professor Dr Dieudonné MUMBA NGOY, a teacher and role model who inspires us enormously. Your comments have shaped us, dear mentor.

To Dr Philippe MASIDI for your sense of reflection, advice and motivation during our time with you, and for drawing up this document.

We would like to thank our brothers and sisters Brave MPIANA, Gédéon MPIANA GEM, Becky MPIANA, Sharon MPIANA, Blaise AMANAKO and my very dear niece Sabdoria Salomé AMANA for your love, support and consideration, which have motivated us and continue to motivate us.

To Pastor Richard DIYOKA, your humility, intelligence and wisdom inspire us to a consecrated life.

To Pastor Paul MPOYI, your humility is an undeniable asset

To Papa Ambroise TSHIYOYO and Mama Nicole SULU, for their infinite consideration, trust and support throughout all this time.

To our beloved brothers and sisters in the Lord Arnold BAYEMBI, Marie KABEDI, Shaloom BOTELE, Roger DISANKA, Eternité BOTELE, Clément MAFUTA and the Germain KALALA family for your advice, prayers and support.

To the Jean MATSHUMBA family for all that you mean to us

To our aunt Léonie BABASENGI receive today our gratitude to you

To the extended family of the Institut National de Recherche Biomédicale (INRB): Dr Nono KUISPOND, Dr Trésor KABEYA, Professeur Papy MANDOKO,Charly KISANGALA,Princesse PAKU,MamanLéontine NKUNKU MBOMA, Dr Nadine MITSEY, Richy BISENGO, Verlaine Moma, Thérèse PEMBE, Gédéon BONGO, Pierrot MULUMBA, Prof Edith NKWEMBE, Dr Lisa LEBO, Andréa MAYUMA, Sandra OISA, Régine KIPOY, Laurette IBANDA, Chimène M, Parfait SHABANI, Alex rex, Ornella MBAYI son excellence, Dido mus, Dr Gilon ILOMBE, Armel TAMFUTU, Mado TSHIYAMBA, Fidélité KALENGAY, Gladis KIKOKO, Marthe SAPATA, Rose BAYEBA, Gloria MISINGI, Lebon MATENDO, for all the moments spent together.

To the MUTOMBE family: Jacquie BOFONDA, Rachel and SALIMA, Michael and Wivine MUTOMBE, Esther MUTOMBE, Matheré EDJOMA, Sam MUTOMBE ;

To Becky MUTOMBE for your consideration and love for us;

To our elders Dr Jephté Bambi NZITA, Dr Agathe NKOY, Dr David NZOLANZO le sanctifié, Dr Guy LUMANDE, Dr Michel LOKANGA, Dr Rosalie KATOKALE, Dr Josué LUMBU, Dr Marc TSHILANDA, Dr Cheffe LIMANGA, Dr Esaïe MUANDA, Dr Bruno BAMPENDE, Dr Gédéon MPURAMANA, you taught us what we needed for our medical training during our internship at the Cliniques Universitaires de Kinshasa.

Loved KUYANGISA a friend and sister, your knowledge is a blessing

To our academic friends who have become a second family, Redy NGALA, Mervedi NTALAKWA, Grace YAMBA, Constance YUMBA, Nathan NSWEYA, Eli TSHISHIMBI, Helene NOUNE, Christian NDONDA, Képhas ZIATA, Daniel

YALE, Jeanne NGONGO, Aimé KUYANGISA Josué NGOMA, Oscar NKULU, Cyril NGIMBI, Parfaite NGITUKA, Fadelish NKETANI, Sarah NGOIE, Priscille NGANGA, Gloria NGOMA, Gradie NGOTOTA, Franck NOGNE, Marie NECHE, Pauline NSAKALA, Stéphane IKPA, Gédéon MANA, Enock MAKUBUKULU, Ezéchiel TADI, Rachel TENGE, Enock LUBAMBA, Félicité SEFU, Laurette MBOMBO, Laetitia NSASA, Eli KAHANGA, for the time spent together.

To dan PULA for the layout of this document

Finally, we would like to thank all those who, from near or far, have contributed to the completion of this work and to the success of our training course.

LIST

SUMMARY

Context: *Smoking is the acute or chronic physiological and psychological intoxication caused tobacco abuse. By extension, the term also refers to tobacco consumption in general. One of the major problems specific to active or passive smoking by women is its impact on their reproductive life. It lengthens the time it takes to conceive, reduces the chances of success of all medically assisted procreation techniques, increases the risk of ectopic pregnancy, spontaneous abortion, low birth weight, sudden infant death syndrome, infectious respiratory and ear, nose and throat diseases and has a harmful effect on the child's overall development.*

Objective: *The aim of this study was to take stock of tobacco consumption among pregnant women receiving antenatal care at the CUK and CHME.*

Methods and results*: This cross-sectional and analytical study on smoking identified 536 pregnant women from two health facilities (FOSA) in the Mont Amba health district of the city of Kinshasa in the DRC. The results showed a smoking rate of 74.4%; 197 pregnant women had at least one previous abortion, 71% of which were spontaneous. The majority of pregnant women had had fewer than three caesarean sections and 40% had experienced two episodes of pre-eclampsia. A history of EP, placenta previa, premature delivery and PMR was found in 6, 7, 4 and 8 pregnant women respectively. The type of tobacco most commonly used was powder; factors associated with smoking were singlehood, secondary education and lack of awareness of the risks associated with smoking. The protective factor against smoking was not drinking alcohol.*

Conclusion and application of results*: Smoking among pregnant women remains high in our environment and therefore constitutes a serious threat to those around them, to the pregnant woman herself and to the product of conception. It is not just the Congolese government that must take responsibility, but everyone, for combating this scourge that threatens our community.*

Key words*: Gestating females, tobacco, consumption, CUK and CHME/Ngaba.*

INTRODUCTION

0.1. Background and justification

Smoking is the acute or chronic physiological and psychological intoxication caused by tobacco abuse (1). By extension, this term also refers to tobacco consumption (2,3). It is sometimes referred to as "active smoking" as opposed to passive smoking, which refers to the involuntary inhalation of tobacco smoke contained in the surrounding air, or the inhalation of secondary airborne deposits (residual smoking) (4).

Smoking is one of the most serious threats ever to global public health. It kills more than 8 million people worldwide every year, including 1.2 million non-smokers involuntarily exposed to smoke (5).

Smoking has been described as "the single most important preventable cause of death in our society and the major public health issue of our time" (6).

One of the major and specific problems of active or passive smoking by women is its impact on their reproductive life, reducing the chances of success of all medically assisted reproduction techniques (MAP), increasing the risk of ectopic pregnancy (EP), spontaneous abortions, low birth weight, sudden infant death syndrome (SIDS), infectious respiratory and otolaryngological pathologies in children and having a harmful effect on their general development (7).

Smoking during pregnancy is the most serious and most frequent form of violence inflicted on the foetus (8). Pregnancy in a woman who uses one or more psychoactive substances (whatever the substance involved) is a high-risk pregnancy. The consequences of psychoactive substance use may be obstetric and/or neonatal (9).

In the USA, around 12% of pregnant women smoke during pregnancy (10), and these rates are even higher among younger women and women of lower socio-economic status, whose children may be more vulnerable than others to developmental problems (10,11).

In France, 22% of pregnant women smoke during pregnancy, which a European record (12). In Africa, the overall rate is low by international standards, with a prevalence rate of 8.4% on the continent. However, the region is one of only two in the world where the WHO predicts an increase in the absolute number of smokers, due to population growth (13). Smoking is a predominantly male habit, and there are substantial differences between the smoking rates of men and women (14).

In the Democratic Republic of Congo (DRC), men consume more tobacco than women. The overall prevalence of tobacco consumption was 26.5% among men and 4.1% among women in 2014 (15).

To the best of our knowledge, to date there has been no study of smoking among pregnant Congolese women, which is why we decided to carry out this study. It will serve as a prelude to further studies on the subject.

0.2. Objectives

0.2.1. General objective

The general aim of this study is to provide overview of the situation of pregnant smokers attending antenatal clinics.

0.2.2. Specific objectives

Our specific objectives are to

- Determining the frequency of smoking among pregnant women
- Identify the socio-demographic situation of women who smoke
- Determine the factors associated with this consumption in our study population

CHAPTER I

GENERAL

1.1. History of tobacco

Tobacco, a simple wild product of a small region of America, remained unknown to the ancient world until 1520, when it was the Spaniards who first stole the plant from the inhabitants of Tabasco, in the province of Yucatan, on the Mexican Sea, in the same country where they had first found the gold of terra firma (16).

The name tobacco they gave it comes both from the place where they discovered it and from tabaccos, certain reeds used by the natives to smoke it. Doctor François Hernandez of Toledo first sent it to Spain and Portugal; a few years later, he perpetuated the name in the Civil and Natural History of America, which he wrote at the behest of Philip II. Some claim that the Spaniards, under the leadership of Columbus, had already found the use established in 1 494 in the large islands where they stopped at the beginning of their discoveries. Magellan's companions were already using it in 1521. From the kingdom of Portugal, tobacco passed to France, where it was brought by Jean Nicot, son of a notary from Nismes (16).

Throughout the ages, tobacco has been known by the following names: ambassadors herb, grand prior's herb, queen's herb (catherinary and medicinal), gentian, holy cross herb, putun, holy herb (16).

Tobacco was used to: treat wounds, in priesthood to render oracles, religious ceremonies (India), incense to make oneself pleasing to the gods (Virginia) (16).

Tobacco was first imported to East Africa by the Portuguese in 1560, before being introduced throughout the continent by the Spanish in 1600 (17).

1.2. Tobacco from a chemical point of view

Tobacco, whose scientific name is Nicotiana tabacum, is a hardy plant in the Solanaceae family, growing from 50 cm to 1.80 metres or more depending on the variety. This annual dicotyledonous plant large leaves, around 30 to 80 cm long and 10 to 40 cm wide. The flower is tubular and coloured at the tip. In the wild, there are around sixty species of tobacco, with nicotine levels ranging from 1 to 10%. The most widely cultivated (90%) is Nicotiana tabacum (18).

1.3. Types of tobacco

Tobacco products include smoked and non-smoked products.

1.3.1. Smoked products

1.3.1.1. Rolling tobacco

Conventional roll-your-own tobacco: higher nicotine, benzene and benzopyrene content than conventional cigarettes
Expanded rolling tobacco: This is tobacco that has been previously impregnated with a highly vaporisable liquid before being placed in an enclosure filled with inert gas (CO2 or liquid nitrogen) and then brutally heated.

1.3.1.2. Blunt

Blunt is made of rolling tobacco leaves made from recomposed raw or flavoured tobacco, with a strong resemblance to a cigar.

1.3.1.3. Cigars and Cigarillos

Cigar smoke contains: more nicotine, carbon monoxide, polycyclic aromatic hydrocarbons and benzene than cigarette smoke: 4 cigars are equivalent to 10 conventional cigarettes (19); A cigarillo is a type of cigar that is small in size, and sometimes the tobacco leaves it contains are chopped into small pieces.

1.3.1.4. Pipe

One pipe is equivalent to 5 cigarettes, according to the Observatoire français des drogues et toxicomanies (OFDT) (20).

1.3.1.5. Hookah (chicha, shisha, water pipe)

The hookah, once used in North Africa and South-East Asia, is growing in popularity in Western countries, particularly among young people. A hookah consists of a glass container half-filled with water, a clay sleeve for the tobacco, a pipe with a valve and a spout. Flavoured tobacco (fruit, various essences) is covered with a sheet of aluminium foil pierced with holes on which a glowing coal is placed. The smoke produced by burning the tobacco in the charcoal passes through the water-filled flask, which cools it. Hookah is smoked by several people over a period of 45 minutes to 1 hour, which is the equivalent of smoking several cigarettes. Although many people think that hookah is less harmful than cigarettes, it is in fact more toxic: the water does not 'filter' the smoke. The levels of tar and aromatic hydrocarbons in the primary stream are at least identical to those of cigarettes, and those of CO and heavy metals are higher in hookah smoke, probably because of the charcoal. The water cools the smoke, leading to deeper inhalation of a volume of more than a litre, whereas a whole cigarette delivers less than a litre of smoke in 15 puffs. Several cases of acute CO poisoning from hookah smoking have been described. Hookah smoking causes the same ailments as cigarettes (respiratory, cardiovascular and cancerous). It can be addictive. The use of a single mouthpiece can be a source of transmission of infectious diseases: herpes, hepatitis, tuberculosis, fungal infections, etc.

1.3.1.6. Heated tobacco :

In many cases they produced more carbon monoxide (CO) than conventional tobacco.

1.3.1.7. Hybrid products

A single capsule contains two components: an e-liquid compartment and a tobacco compartment.

1.3.1.8. Bidis

These cigarettes are very common in Asia and the Middle East, and have the particularity of being flavoured with fruit or chocolate.

1.3.1.9. Kretek

These cigarettes are made in Indonesia and flavoured with cloves.

1.3.1.10. Electronic cigarette

Its vapour contains propylene glycol, an irritant solvent whose long-term effects are poorly understood. However, a toxicological study of electronic cigarettes published in New Zealand in 2008 (Ruyan products) reported no short-term health effects, apart from pharyngeal irritation.

1.3.2. Unsmoked tobacco

1.3.1.11. Snuff or taking

Snuff is made from finely chopped, dried tobacco leaves and comes in the form of ground tobacco for nasal inhalation**.** The nicotine in snuff is absorbed through the mucous membranes of the nose and can cause dependence. The rate of absorption is rapid, comparable to cigarette smoke, and increases when the pH of the tobacco is alkaline. In addition to nicotine, snuff contains carcinogenic substances such as nitrosamines.

1.3.1.12. Chewing tobacco

Mouthing tobacco is as old as the discovery of the product on the Old Continent.

1.3.1.13. Chique

The product is a firm substance resulting from the crumbling and agglomeration of tobacco leaves in various forms.

1.3.1.14. Vaginal tobacco

The substance, described as a "miracle" because it allows you "send your man to 7th heaven", is made from dried tobacco leaves and the roots a tree named "tangora" or other plants such as "kankouran mano" or "koundinding". We also have **soluble smokeless tobacco, toothpaste and tobacco water.**

1.4. Composition of cigarette smoke

Cigarette smoke is an aerosol that mixes gases and particles. It contains around 4,000 different substances, 40 of which are carcinogenic (21). The four main components are **nicotine**, **carbon monoxide**, **irritant compounds and tars**

(22). When cigarettes are lit, combustion leads to the formation of numerous toxic compounds such as tar, various toxic gases (carbon monoxide, nitrogen oxide, hydrocyanic acid, ammonia), heavy metals (cadmium, lead, chromium, mercury) and irritants (23).

1.4.1. Nicotine

It is the best-known component of cigarettes. It is implicated in tobacco dependence, which appears after the first few weeks of exposure and at low levels of consumption. However, it is thought to result from the interaction between several substances. Monoamine oxidase inhibitors (MAOIs), for example, appear to play an important role in the addictive potential of nicotine (24). Nicotine reaches the brain in 9 to 19 seconds (faster than after an intravenous injection) and reaches a peak after 20 to 30 minutes. Its elimination half-life is around two hours (20). It binds to nicotinic cholinergic receptors and stimulates reward systems by modulating the release of numerous neurotransmitters.

1.4.2. Carbon monoxide (CO)

Is a gas formed when cigarettes are burnt. Its toxicity is due to its high affinity with the haemoglobin molecule. Once attached to haemoglobin, CO has a stronger affinity than oxygen for the iron in haemoglobin, causing hypoxia as a result of a lack of oxygen transport. The body then responds with tachycardia and increased blood pressure, leading to increased cardiac risk.

1.4.3. Tars

These are the compounds mainly implicated in the development of cancers linked to cigarette smoking. This generic term encompasses a large number of different molecules: hydrocarbons such as benzene and benzopyrene, which is carcinogenic because of its properties as a deoxyribonucleic acid (DNA) intercalating agent.

1.4.4. Chronic exposure

Heavy metals, such as lead or cadmium, can :

- Causes problems in the bones of the skeleton by substituting for calcium in bone crystals;
- Lead to lung cancer;
- Induce kidney damage, the toxicity of which is caused by chronic exposure and the syndromes of which are well known. These heavy metals are present in large varieties, forming a toxic "cocktail" that accumulates over time.

1.4.5. Irritating substances

Nitrosamines are highly carcinogenic. Inhaling acrolein causes a burning sensation, coughing, sore throats, nausea... These substances encourage the production of thickened mucus (21). Tobacco smoke also contains phenols, hydrocyanic acid and other aldehydes that can be classified as irritants.

1.4.6. Additives

Flavourings are used for a variety of reasons, including to give cigarette a particular flavour in order to build brand loyalty. Flavouring cigarettes also helps to mask bitterness or unpleasant odours, sweeten the smoke and reduce airway irritation. Additives also help control the way the cigarette burns and maintain constant humidity to prevent the tobacco from becoming dry. They can also be used to whiten smoke and ash to improve the overall appearance of the cigarette and make its image more attractive. The lack of any real knowledge of what additives produce during combustion or of their intrinsic and collective toxicity poses a problem (22). For example, acetaldehyde, a substance produced by the breakdown of ethanol in the body, is used as a flavouring agent and is produced by the combustion of many molecules, such as sorbitol and glycerol. It is one of the main components cigarette smoke. The problem with acetaldehyde is its high reactivity. It is classified as a possible human carcinogen by the International Agency for Research on Cancer (IARC) and is also irritating to the respiratory tract. It would appear that this substance increases dependence on cigarettes and potentiates dependence on nicotine. One of its breakdown products, harmane, is thought to have an antidepressant effect, inhibiting monoamine oxidase, which is indirectly involved in cigarette addiction.

1.5. Metabolism

Tobacco smoke acts directly or indirectly on almost every organ in the body. The toxic products are deposited on the mucous membranes of the mouth, larynx, lungs and oesophagus, and the gaseous components and microparticles carried by the blood exert their harmful effects on the arteries and various organs (25,26).

1.5.1. Active smoking

Three smoke streams are formed:

- **Primary**, which represents the smoke released as soon as the smoker "pulls" on the cigarette;
- **Secondary**, which is the smoke that comes out of the end of the cigarette;
- **Tertiary**, which is equivalent to the proportion of smoke inhaled by the smoker that is released during the next exhalation.

The composition of smoke varies more according to the smoking method than the brand and type of cigarette. Second-hand smoke contains a particularly high concentration of toxic products (25). These toxic particles then penetrate different parts of the body depending on their diameter. The largest remain in the upper airways where, in direct contact with the mucous membranes, they can cause irritation, increasing the incidence of ear, nose and throat (ENT) diseases, and impair the purification system (thicker mucus, inhibited ciliary movements). They therefore remain in contact with the body for longer, which increases their harmful long-term effects. The finest particles reach the lower airways, the alveoli, where they enter the blood, which carries them via the arteries to all the body's organs. Because they penetrate the various sites of the body, the complications of active smoking are numerous. Tobacco remains the most important risk factor in lung cancer.

1.5.2. Passive smoking

Passive smoking is defined as the involuntary inhalation of tobacco smoke released into atmosphere by one or more smokers (24). Non-smokers inhale the secondary current and a tiny part of the tertiary current. As well as causing discomfort, passive smoking aggravates existing illnesses and can create new ones. The World Health Organisation (WHO) estimates that passive smoking causes 603,000 deaths a year worldwide, or 1% of global mortality. Complications affect those around the smoker, especially young children.

Nicotine enters the bloodstream through the use and handling of tobacco products and exposure to second-hand smoke. When nicotine reaches the liver, kidneys and lungs, it is metabolised into a number of main breakdown products known as cotinine, cotinine-N-glucuronide, nicotine-N-glucuronide, trans-3'-hydroxycotinine and trans-3-hydroxycotinine-O-glucuronide (27). Together with nicotine itself, these breakdown products (metabolites) are specific biomarkers of exposure to tobacco whose concentration in urine or blood can be measured. This data can then be used to determine a person's level of exposure to tobacco products or tobacco smoke. (28)

Cotinine is one of the most effective biomarkers of exposure to tobacco products and tobacco smoke. (29) It can easily be measured in urine or blood (30,31) and can be detected in the body up to four days after exposure to nicotine (32,33). Cotinine is specific to nicotine and provides a reliable measure of exposure to tobacco products and tobacco smoke. The cotinine assay has recently been successfully used to validate self-reported smoking habits. (34)

Tobacco consumption can have a major impact on the effect of certain medicines. The polycyclic aromatic hydrocarbons produced when tobacco and cigarette paper are burnt induce the activity of a number of proteins, including an isoform of the cytochrome P450 family, cytochrome P450 1A2 (CYP1A2). This induction can reduce the plasma levels of drugs metabolised by this isoform, and consequently their efficacy.4 Conversely, when smoking is stopped, the plasma concentration of these drugs can sometimes reach toxic levels, necessitating a reduction in the dose administered.4 This review therefore proposes to address the various genetic aspects of smoking and smoking cessation, as well as recommendations for the management of patients taking certain drugs when they stop smoking.

1.6. The effect of tobacco a woman's body

In addition to the well-known consequences of smoking for human beings, we note in particular for women:

1.6.1. Female fertility

Active smoking is statistically significantly associated with a delay in conception independent of tubal infertility factors. A dose-response relationship and reversibility when smoking is stopped have been demonstrated. This risk has also been suggested for passive smoking (35). In medically assisted reproduction (MAP), maternal smoking is significantly associated with a reduction in oocyte collection and possibly in the implantation rate. The effects are all the more marked when the partner is a smoker.

Smoking is also significantly associated with an increase in the age of menopause (2 years on average). This phenomenon is all the more pronounced the more cigarettes are smoked and for longer. But it is partially reversible. The fertility of daughters exposed in utero to their mother's smoking habits is also statistically significantly reduced.

The pathophysiological hypotheses put forward to explain the tobacco-related reduction in female fertility are :

- The endocrine action of nicotine is antiestrogenic, with a particular effect on cervical mucus;
- Tobacco derivatives have a direct toxic effect on the ovary;
- Changes in the ciliary function of the fallopian tubes (35).

1.6.2. Ectopic pregnancies

Smoking is statistically significantly associated with an increased risk of EP (around 35% of EPs are attributable to smoking). A dose-response relationship and partial reversibility have been found.

Experimental studies in animals and in vitro suggest a plausible pathophysiological mechanism:

- Decreased ciliary beat ;
- Impaired tubal contractility ;
- Impaired adhesion of the oocyte to the tubal pinna (35).

1.6.3. Spontaneous abortions

Several studies have shown a statistically significant increase in the risk of spontaneous abortion in both active and passive smokers (35).

1.7. Effect of tobacco on the product of conception and the course of pregnancy

1.7.1. Tobacco and malformations

Tobacco does not have a significant teratogenic effect, since it does not increase the overall frequency of malformations, which is 2 to 3% in the human species.

On the other hand, smoking during organogenesis (1st trimester) increases the occurrence of certain specific malformations. It should be noted that most of these anomalies are rare in the general population, and that the increased risk associated with smoking does little to increase their number in absolute terms. Furthermore, studies did not take into account other risk factors for malformations (alcohol, co-addictions, nutritional status).

- Facial clefts
- Craniostenosis
- Other malformations: neural tube closure anomalies, cardiac malformations

and hypospadias (35).

1.7.2. Retroplacental haematoma

Eight studies have shown a statistically significant relationship between smoking and the occurrence of retroplacental haematoma (RPH), with 25% of RPHs linked to smoking. The higher the serum carboxyhaemoglobin (HbCO) level, the greater the risk of PRH, and the greater the risk with age and parity.

The occurrence of smoking-related HRP is explained by the vasoconstrictive effect of tobacco products (including nicotine) and the increase in capillary fragility (35).

1.7.3. Low inserted placenta

The risk of a low-lying placenta is multiplied by 2 if a pregnant woman smokes. A dose-response relationship has been demonstrated in a single study (35).

1.7.4. Prematurity

This prematurity is largely due to the more frequent occurrence of obstetric accidents (HRP, low-lying placenta with haemorrhage or premature rupture of the membranes). The proportion of prematurity due to maternal hypertension appears to be lower in smokers. Smoking cessation before conception or during the 1st trimester reduces the risk for the current pregnancy and subsequent pregnancies (20).

1.7.5. Premature rupture of the membranes

Smoking during pregnancy is associated with a doubling of the risk of premature rupture of the membranes, especially in the case of very premature births. A dose-response relationship has not been demonstrated. The mechanism suggested is a stimulation of PGE2, which causes uterine contractions, and an increase in bacterial vaginosis in pregnant smokers (35).

1.7.6. Intrauterine growth retardation

Smoking during pregnancy is a proven risk factor for intrauterine growth retardation (IUGR). The average weight deficit is 200 grams. This is a harmonious IUGR (weight, height and head circumference below the tenth percentile), with greater emphasis on muscle mass.

The pathophysiological mechanism of IUGR linked to smoking is probably multifactorial, resulting in particular from: chronic hypoxia; uterine and umbilical vasoconstriction; cadmium toxicity; undernourishment of pregnant smokers (35).

1.7.7. Brain development

The reduction in head circumference at birth is statistically significantly associated with maternal smoking, with a dose-response relationship. This reduction raises fears of inadequate prenatal brain development, particularly when the reduction is greater than or equal to 15-20 mm. In addition to the effects of hypoxia, direct biochemical toxicity of nicotine on foetal brain development has been reported in several animal studies (35).

1.7.8. Foetal death in utero

Maternal smoking is associated with an excess of foetal deaths during the 3rd trimester. These in utero deaths are not linked solely to IUGR or placental complications; the permanent stimulation of nicotine receptors in the brain involved in the control of breathing and sleep on the one hand, and cardiomyopathy on the other, could expose the foetus to the risk of sudden death in utero (35).

1.7.9. Foetal well-being

Maternal smoking has an impact on the overall well-being of the foetus during pregnancy, as it leads to :

- chronic hypoxia: chronic hypoxia is a key factor in altering foetal well-being. It results from the interplay of various factors: formation of HbCO under the effect of CO; uteroplacental vasoconstriction induced by nicotine peaks and/or the oxidising substances in cigarette smoke; placental anomalies (HRP, low-insert placenta); foetal cardiovascular repercussions of nicotine;
- cardiovascular repercussions: the immediate response to maternal inhalation of

cigarette smoke is an increase in heart rate and output and vasoconstriction;

- respiratory repercussions: the rhythm of foetal respiratory movements is altered following inhalation of cigarette smoke. Smoking disrupts lung growth, leads to bronchial hyperreactivity and increased cellular permeability to antigens, with increased IgE levels in cord blood;
- a reduction in foetal movements: chronic exposure to tobacco in utero is accompanied by an overall reduction in foetal movements (35).

CHAPTER II

MATERIALS AND METHODS

2.1. Type and period of study

This is a cross-sectional and analytical study carried out over a period running from 03 May to 29 September 2023.

2.2. Study framework

2.2.1. Choice of frame

The study took place at the Cliniques Universitaires de Kinshasa and the Centre Hospitalier Mère et Enfants de Ngaba.

2.2.2. Description

The CUK is located on the Campus of the University of Kinshasa (UNIKIN) on the Mont-Amba hill in the Commune of Lemba. This university hospital was set up in 1957 to provide health care for the population, teach medicine and paramedical sciences, and carry out medical research. The CUK is under the triple supervision of the Ministries of Higher and University Education, Health and Research. It has a capacity of 565 beds and has expertise in all the medical fields and specialities available in the DRC.

The CHME/Ngaba is a General Reference Hospital in Ngaba, located in the Commune of Ngaba on Avenue KIANZA N°58, in the MOKULUA district. The hospital opened its doors in 1991 and has continued to develop and diversify its medical capabilities, providing ever greater care for an increasingly impoverished population. It is also very active in public health research (AIDS, sickle cell anaemia, malaria) and the training of health professionals.

2.3. Sampling

2.3.1. Patients

The sample was exhaustive and comprised 536 pregnant animals, which were selected on the basis of the criteria below.

2.3.2. Selection criteria

All pregnant women attending the above-mentioned health facilities during the study period were included after obtaining informed consent. They were selected from the active file.

Any pregnant woman who did not give her consent was not included.

2.4. Data collection

2.4.1. Data collection tool

The data was collected using a pre-established form, shown in the appendix. It contained three sectionsgeneral characteristics, gynaecological and obstetric history, cardiovascular risk factors and lifestyle.

2.4.2. Data collection technique

The data were collected by structured interview. The first stage consisted of explaining the purpose of the study to the pregnant women, and in the second stage, the participants were asked to complete the pre-established questionnaire.

2.5.Variables of interest

2.5.1. General characteristics

- Age ;
- Profession ;
- Home address (district) ;
- Level of education ;
- Province of origin ;
- Religion.

2.5.2. Gynaecological and obstetrical characteristics

- Gestité
- Parity

- Abortion

2.5.3. Characteristics related to tobacco consumption

- Smoking: was defined as tobacco consumption by the pregnant women themselves (active smoking) or by other household members (passive smoking).
- Frequency of smoking ;
- Type of tobacco ;
- Period of pregnancy during which she is exposed to tobacco ;
- Reason for smoking ;
- Risk awareness ;
- Acceptance or otherwise of withdrawal in pregnant smokers.

2.6. Data processing and analysis

The data collected was checked before being compiled and analysed on an HP brand computer using SPSS version 26.0 software. Word processing and the preparation of tables and graphs were carried out using Microsoft WORD and EXCEL version 2016.

Categorical variables are presented as frequency and proportion, and continuous quantitative variables as mean, standard deviation and extremes. Our results are summarised in the tables and figures.

Fischer's exact test was used to compare proportions and logistic regression was used to search for associated factors. The significance threshold was set at a p-value <0.05.

2.7. Ethical considerations

The data was collected confidentially and processed anonymously. All participants gave their informed consent before the interview. We obtained a letter of authorisation from the Medical Directors of the CUK and the CHME/Ngaba before collecting the data. There were no conflicts of interest in this study.

CHAPTER III

RESULTS

3.1. Descriptive epidemiology

3.1.1. Frequency of smoking

Figure 1 shows the frequency of smoking among pregnant women undergoing ANC in the two health facilities. It shows that 74.4% of pregnant women were smokers.

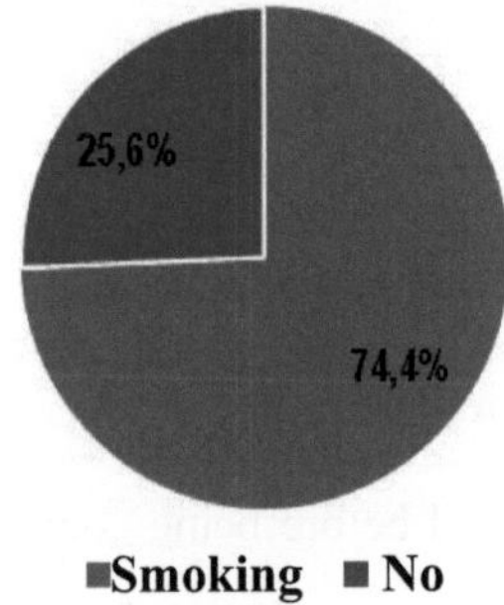

Figure 1 : Frequency of smoking among pregnant women followed in ANC

3.1.2. Type of smoking

The figure below defines the smoking categories, showing that passive smoking accounted for 83.7% of pregnant women.

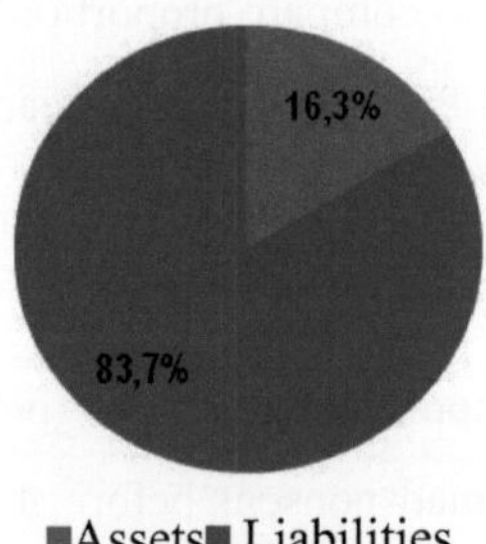

Figure 2: Breakdown of pregnant women by smoking status

3.1.3. General characteristics of pregnant women

Table I summarises the general characteristics of the pregnant animals.

Pregnant women attending the CHME, pregnant women living in the Mont Amba district, married women, housewives and pregnant women with secondary education were more exposed to smoking than others. This difference was statistically significant. There was no statistically significant relationship between age and religion in relation to smoking.

Table I: Distribution of patients according to general characteristics of pregnant women

Variable Population Smoking p

	n=536	Yes (n=399)	No (n=137)	
FOSA CUK	221(41,2)	138(34,6)	83(60,6)	<0,001*
CHME Ngaba	315(58,8)	261(65,4)	54(39,4)	
Age < 18 years old	10(1,9)	10(2,5)	0(00)	0,172
18 - 34 years old	387(72,2)	287(71,9)	100(73)	
≥ 35 years old	139(25,9)	102(25,6)	37(27)	
Place of residence Mount Amba	335(62,5)	257(64,4)	78(56,9)	0,021*
Lukunga	98(18,3)	62(15,5)	36(26,3)	
Funa	89(16,6)	70(17,5)	19(13,9)	
Tshangu	14(2,6)	10(2,5)	4(2,9)	
Civil status Single	129(24,1)	108(27,1)	21(15,3)	0,008*
Married	406(75,7)	290(72,7)	116(84,7)	
Divorced	1(0,2)	1(0,2)	0	
Profession Employee	171(31,9)	110(27,6)	61(44,5)	<0,001*
Housekeeper	241(45)	200(50,1)	41(29,9)	
Liberal	94(17,5)	66(16,5)	28(20,4)	
Unemployed	30(5,6)	23(5,8)	7(5,1)	
Level of education Primary	10(1,9)	9(2,3)	1(0,7)	0,001*

Secondary	285(53,2)	230(57,6)	55(40,1)	
University	233(43,5)	154(38,6)	79(57,7)	
Professional	2(0,4)	1(0,3)	1(0,7)	
Religion Church of revival	218(40,7)	158(39,6)	60(43,8)	0,271
Catholic	193(36)	146(36,6)	47(34,3)	
Protestant	84(15,7)	59(14,8)	25(18,2)	
Kimbanguist	28(5,2)	24(6)	4(2,9)	
Islam	13(2,4)	12(3)	1(0,6)	

3.1.4. Province origin

Table II shows the provinces of origin of the pregnant women interviewed. As a result, the majority of pregnant women who took part in our study were from central Kongo (16%). There was no significant association between province and smoking (p=0.327).

Table II: Breakdown of patients by province of origin

Province	All		Smoking	
	n=536	Yes (n=399)		No (n=137)
Bas Uele	4(0,7)	3(0,8)		1(0,7)
Ecuador	39(7,3)	32(8,1)		7(5,1)
Haut Katanga	10(1,9)	8(2,0)		2(1,5)
Upper Lomami	2(0,4)	2(0,5)		0(0,0)
Upper Uele	4(0,7)	2(0,5)		2(1,5)
Ituri	7(1,3)	6(1,6)		1(0,7)
Central Kasai	33(6,2)	25(6,3)		8(5,8)
Kasai Oriental	70(13,1)	47(11,8)		23(16,8)
Kongo Central	86(16,0)	64(16,0)		22(16,1)
Kwango	30(5,6)	23(5,8)		7(5,1)
Kwilu	82(15,3)	63(15,8)		19(13,9)
Lomami	17(3,2)	12(3,0)		5(3,6)
Lualaba	9(1,7)	7(1,8)		2(1,5)
Maindombe	22(4,1)	14(3,5)		8(5,8)
Maniema	12(2,2)	9(2,3)		3(2,2)
Mongala	23(4,3)	17(4,3)		6(4,4)
North Kivu	17(3,2)	12(3,1)		5(3,7)
North Ubangi	3(0,6)	1(0,3)		2(1,5)
Sankuru	23(4,3)	19(4,8)		4(2,9)

South Kivu	10(1,9)	7(1,8)		3(2,2)
South Ubangi	6(1,1)	4(1,0)		2(1,5)
Tanganyika	11(2,1)	8(2,0)		3(2,2)
Tshopo	5(0,9)	5(1,3)		0(00)
Tshuapa	9(1,7)	7(1,8)		2(1,5)
Cameroon	2(0,4)	2(0,5)		0(00)

3.1.5. Clinic

3.1.5.1. Gynaecological and obstetrical history

Tables IIIa, IIIb and IIIc summarise the gynaecological and obstetrical characteristics of the patients. From Tables IIIa and IIIb, it can be seen that gynaecological-obstetrical history was significantly associated with smoking.

Table IIIa. Gynaeco-obstetrical history

Variable Population Smoking p

	n=536	Yes n=399	No n=137	
Parity 0	150(28)	113(28,3)	37(27)	0,257
1	126(25,5)	100(25,1)	26(19)	
≥ 2	260(48,5)	186(46,6)	74(54)	
Gestité 1	155(28,9)	119(29,8)	36(26,3)	0,447
≥ 2	381(71,1)	280(70,2)	101(73,7)	
Abortion Yes	197(36,8)	150(37,6)	47(34,3)	0,439
No	339(63,2)	249(62,4)	90(65,7)	
Caesarean section history Yes	88(16,4)	72(18)	16(11,7)	0,271
No	448(83,6)	327(82)	121(88,3)	
HISTORY OF MISCARRIAGE Yes	6(1,1)	5(1,3)	1(0,7)	0,520
No	530(98,9)	394(98,7)	136(99,3)	
Pregnancy (SA) < 28	359(67,1)	269(67,4)	90(65,7)	0,258
28 - 36	144(26,9)	110(27,6)	34(24,8)	
≥ 37	32(6)	20(5)	13(9,5)	

Table IIIb. Gynaeco-obstetrical history

Variable	Population	Smoking		p
	n=536	Yes	No	
Current pre-eclampsia Yes	4(0,7)	3(0,8)	1(0,7)	0,842
No	532(99,3)	396(99,2)	136(99,3)	
History of pre-eclampsia Yes	25(4,7)	19(4,8)	6(4,4)	0,938
No	511(95,3)	380(95,2)	131(95,6)	
Placenta previa Yes	7(1,3)	6(1,5)	1(0,7)	0,866
No	529(98,7)	393(98,5)	136(99,3)	
Premature delivery Yes	4(0,7)	2(0,5)	2(1,5)	0,458
No	532(99,3)	397(99,5)	135(98,5)	
RPM Yes	8(1,5)	7(1,8)	1(0,7)	0,906
No	528(98,5)	392(98,2)	136(99,3)	
MAR Yes	155(28,9)	119(29,8)	36(26,3)	0,803
No	381(71,1)	280(70,2)	101(73,7)	
IUGR Yes	3(0,6)	3(0,8)	0(0,0)	0,820
No	533(99,4)	396(99,2)	137(100)	

Table IIIc shows that 197 pregnant women had at least one previous abortion, 71% of which were spontaneous. The majority of pregnant women had had fewer than three caesarean sections; 83% had been hypertensive for less than five years and 40% had had two episodes of pre-eclampsia. A history of EP, placenta previa, premature delivery and PMR was found in 6, 7, 4 and 8 pregnant women respectively.

Table IIIc. Gynaeco-obstetrical history

Variable	Population	%
Type abortion Spontaneous	n=197 139	 70,6
Provoked	58	29,4
Number of caesarean sections < 3	n=88 80	 90,9
≥ 3	8	9,1
Duration of hypertension < 5 years	n=18 15	 83,3
≥ 5 years	3	16,7
Number of cases of pre-eclampsia A	n=25 15	 60
Two	10	40
Variable	Population	Proportion
Number of EPs A	n=6 4	 4/6
Two	2	2/6
Number of Placenta previa < 2	n=7 6	 6/7
≥ 2	1	1/7
Number premature deliveries A	n=4 4	 4/4
RPM A	n=8 8	 8/8

3.2. Smoking-related characteristics

The incidence of active smoking was 16.3%.

3.2.1. Type of tobacco

The table below shows the types of tobacco used by pregnant women. Powdered tobacco was the most commonly used type of tobacco, consumed alone in 55% of cases, with cigarettes in 10.8% and with shisha in 7.7%.

Table IV. Type of tobacco

Type of tobacco	n=65	%
In powder form	48	73,8
Only	36	55,4
Cigarette	7	10,8
Shisha	5	7,7
Cigarette	17	26,2
Only	14	21,5
Shisha	3	4,6

3.2.2. Alcohol and tobacco consumption habits

The table below shows the characteristics according to alcohol and tobacco consumption. Most of the 162 pregnant women who consumed alcohol were smokers; we found that pregnant women who smoked also usually consumed alcohol.

Table V. Alcohol and tobacco consumption

Variable	Population	Smoking		p
	n=536	Yes n=399	No n=137	
Alcohol Yes	162(30,2)	143(35,8)	19(13,9)	<0,001
No	374(67,8)	256(64,2)	118(86,1)	

3.2.2.1. Duration of alcohol consumption

The figure below shows the duration of alcohol consumption. It can be seen that the majority of pregnant women had been drinking alcohol for < 5 years.

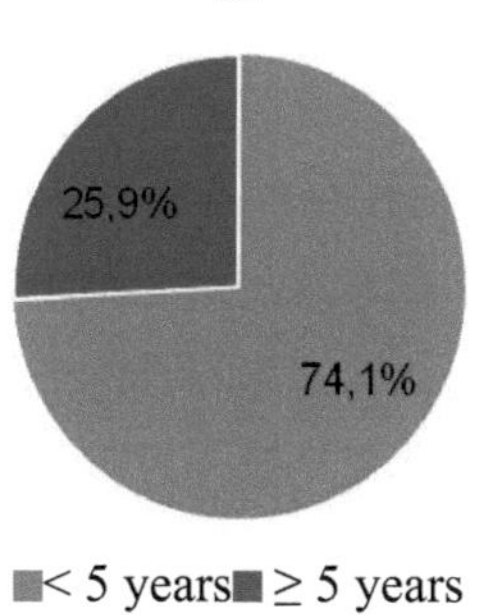

■< 5 years■ ≥ 5 years

Figure 3. Duration of alcohol consumption

3.2.2.2. Duration of smoking

The table below shows the duration smoking by pregnant women. It can be seen from the table below that the duration of smoking was between 3-5 years, with 49.2% of pregnant smokers being active smokers.

Table VI. Duration of actual smoking

Duration of smoking	n=65	%
< 1 year	7	10,8
1 - 3 years	21	32,3
3 - 5 years	32	49,2
> 5 years	5	7,7

3.2.2.3. Daily smoking frequency

Table VII shows the daily frequency of smoking

Nearly five out of 10 pregnant women smoked more than three times a day.

Table VII. Daily smoking frequency

Daily smoking frequency	n=65	%
<3	20	30,8
3	11	16,9
>3	32	49,2
Imprecise	2	3,1

Risks associated with smoking

The table below shows pregnant women's knowledge of the risks associated with smoking The majority of smokers were unaware of the risks associated with smoking compared with others. This difference was significant.

Table VIII. Awareness of smoking-related risks

Variable	Population	Smoking		p
	n=536	Yes n=399	No n=137	
Knowledge Yes	67(12,5)	40(10)	27(19,7)	<0,004
No	469(87,5)	359(9	110(80,3)	

The table below shows the risks of smoking cited by pregnant women. Abortion and primiparity were the most well-known risks of smoking in 90.8% and 35% respectively.

Table IX. Risks of smoking

Risk of smoking	n	%
Abortion	59	90,8
Prematurity	23	35,4
IUGR	7	10,8
Preeclampsia	1	1,5

3.2.2.4. Attitude to smoking cessation

Figure 3 shows the smoking cessation rate among pregnant smokers. The majority of smokers were in favour of cessation.

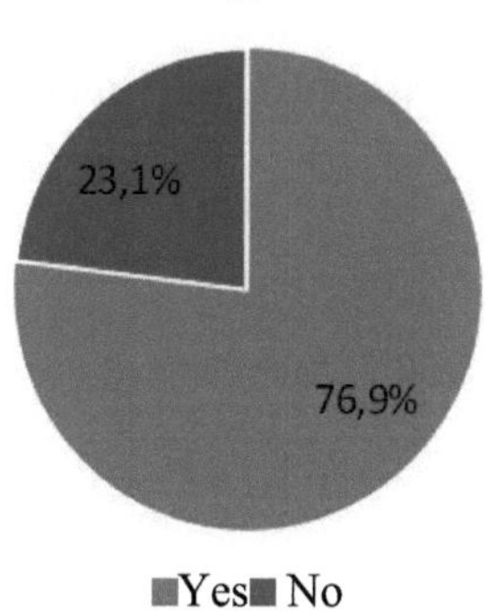

Figure 4: Smoking cessation

3.3. Analytical epidemiology

3.3.1. Factors associated with smoking

The factors associated with smoking were singlehood, secondary education, ignorance of the risks of smoking and not drinking alcohol. The first three factors significantly increased the likelihood of smoking, while not drinking alcohol was a protective factor against smoking, as shown in the table below.

Table X: Factors associated with tobacco consumption

Variable	p	OR	CI (95%)
District of residence Mount amba	0,648	1,3	(0,402 - 4,319)
Lukunga	0,553	0,7	0,201 - 2,357
Funa	0,548	1,5	(0,416 - 5,224)
Tshangu	1	1	
Civil status Single	0,006*	2,1	(1,230 - 3,442)
Divorced	-	-	-
Married	1	1	
Profession Employee	0,192	0,5	(0,223 - 1,353)
Liberal	0,495	0,7	(0,276 - 1,863)
Housekeeper	0,395	1,5	(0,597 - 3,690)
Unemployed	1	1	
Level of education Primary	0,150	4,6	(0,575 - 37,093)
Secondary	<0,001*	2,1	(1,438 - 3,201)
Professional	0,603	1,5	(0,304 - 7,801)
University	1	1	
Alcohol No	<0,001*	0,3	(0,168 - 0,480)
Yes	1	1	
Knowledge of tobacco-related risks			
No	0,004*	2,2	(1,293 - 3,753)
Yes	1	1	

CHAPTER IV

DISCUSSION

4.1. Frequency of smoking

The prevalence of smoking among pregnant women remains a cause for concern. Despite the risks during this precious period, many pregnant women continue to smoke (36). Worldwide, the prevalence of active smoking among pregnant women was estimated at 25% in 2009 (37). Our study found a frequency of 74.4%, which is very high compared with that reported in the North American territories, with a frequency of 59.3% (38). Our prevalence of active smoking is close to those found respectively in the USA in 2010 and Canada in 2013 at 10.7% and 23.3% (39). We found a very high frequency of passive smoking compared to that found between July 2003 and June 2004 in France where 55% of pregnant women were exposed to passive smoking (40). the same finding was made in 4 regions of Spain in 2013 (41).Protecting pregnant women from secondary exposure must be a key maternal and child health strategy (40).

4.2. General characteristics

4.2.1. Age

The mean age in our study was 29.8 years; the same age was found in France in 2010 by Maïté BRU (42). In our study, the 18-34 age group represented the majority of pregnant smokers, probably similar to that found in the above study (42). In fact, it is not the fact of being in this age group that forces pregnant women to be smokers, but rather the majority of our sample was in this age group and it is also the period when fertility is at its highest. The youngest woman in our study was 12 years oldwhich is why it is so important to protect pregnant women and the products they use to conceive their babies.

4.2.2. Civil status

Married women made up the majority of smokers, and the same observation was made in France in 2010 (42). In our study, single pregnant women who abused tobacco were very considerable because they were influenced by the environment around them.

4.2.3. Profession

In our study we found that the majority of pregnant women were housewives; this occupation differs from that reported in Limoge in 2022, where the majority pregnant smokers were employed (43).

Our study shows that there is no statistically significant link between smoking and occupation. Although the majority were housewives, this can be explained by the precarious situation that reigns in our environment, with unemployment at an all-time high in our society, where almost the entire population lives on less than one US dollar a day.

4.2.4. Level of education

In our study we found that the majority of pregnant women had secondary education. This can be explained by the fact that in the study region the financial conditions of the population remain poor.

4.2.5. Province origin

The province of Central Kongo was the most represented. This can be explained by the fact that the population living in the vicinity of the study site originates from the province of Central Kongo.

4.3. Gynaecological and obstetric history

Multiparity was the predominant gynaeco-obstetrical status in our study, which is different from what was found in Limoge in 2022, where more primiparous women were involved (43); In the DRC, the average household size is 9, and most households live in communal courtyards, which exposes pregnant women more to passive smoking.

4.4. Smoking habits

4.4.1. Risk awareness

Of the known risks, abortion and prematurity were the most frequently cited; in France in 2014, respiratory problems and growth retardation the most frequently reported (44). The more pregnant women knew about the risks of smoking, the less they smoked and the more they gave up smoking for fear of harming their unborn child.

4.4.2. Consumer motivation

Most of the pregnant women interviewed in our study cited pleasure, getting rid of worries and treating sinusitis as the reasons for smoking. The literature highlights the bad habit women have of using powdered tobacco intra-vaginally to boost libidinal energy. The substance is said to be a 'miracle' because it can 'send your man to 7th heaven'.

4.4.3. Types of tobacco used

Figures for the prevalence of substance use during pregnancy are unknown in France and are probably underestimated in the rest of the world, as studies have generally used questionnaires rather than assays (45).

The most commonly used tobacco products in France in 2014 were electronic cigarettes (vapoteuse), snus, chicha (46)

In our study, we found that powdered tobacco was consumed either alone or in combination with cigarettes and/or shisha.

In our society today, there is one phenomenon that is beating the record, and that is the use of chicha, which is much more toxic than cigarettes (47).

4.4.4. Factors associated with smoking

The factors reported in the literature singlehoodmaternal age under 20 and unemployment (48). In our study, apart from singlehood, we also ignorance of the risks associated with smoking and secondary education. In France in 2020, it was reported that maternal age over 34 years was a protective factor against smoking (48); whereas in our study, the absence of alcohol consumption was a protective factor.

4.4.5. Attitude to withdrawal

In France, the absence of smoking cessation during pregnancy is associated with low socio-economic status (48). This finding may be explained by low socio-economic status, as cessation requires the means to purchase certain substitutes. According to a meta-analysis carried out in France in 2020, 76.2% of pregnant smokers accepted cessation (48); this is similar to that found in our study, where 76.9% of pregnant smokers accepted cessation.

Smoking addiction is a serious and chronic disease. Even after quitting, smokers will never be safe from a relapse, particularly after giving birth, returning home or taking postnatal leave. Dealing with this addiction is at the heart of prenatal care for mothers and fathers-to-be. The mobilisation of midwives and other perinatal professionals can contribute to better control of smoking.

CONCLUSION

The aim of our study was to assess smoking among pregnant women receiving antenatal care at the CUK and CME/Ngaba. It revealed that 74.4% of pregnant women in our sample smoked during their pregnancy, with 83.7% being passive smokers; Our study shows that 35.8% of women who smoked also consumed alcohol. The factors associated with smoking were singlehood, secondary education, lack of awareness of the risks of smoking and not consuming alcohol, while not consuming alcohol was a protective factor against smoking. Pregnancy is a key time for adopting the best lifestyle habits, particularly giving up smoking, and deterrence strategies are an asset in the fight against this scourge.

RECOMMENDATIONS

❖ **Ministry of Health (DRC) :**

- Instruct all tobacco product manufacturers to display a pictogram on tobacco product packaging;
- Organise comprehensive awareness campaigns in the health zones with the help of community relays, who are very close to the community;
- Improve anti-smoking messages to the point where they are not a condemnation but a help pregnant women.

❖ **Healthcare professionals:**

- Make pregnant women aware of the dangers of active and passive smoking during ANC;
- Helping pregnant women with practices to be applied in event of secondary or tertiary exposure to tobacco smoke

❖ **Pregnant women**:

- Follow and put into practice the advice received healthcare staff on how to lead a happy life.
- secondary and tertiary exposure to tobacco smoke

❖ **Family and friends :**

- up smoking, because second-hand and third-hand smoke is harmful to her health, and to that of the pregnant woman in particular.
- Protect pregnant women from all products.

REFERENCES

1. Quillet medical encyclopaedia, "Tabagisme" [archive], on Analyse et traitement informatique de la langue française, 1965.

2. Tabac : la consommation repart à la hausse" [archive], on Le Figaro, 19 October 2010 (accessed 29 May 2017)

3. Smoking and health" [archive], in Gouvernement du Québec (consulted on 29 May 2017)

4. "The social image of tobacco", on inpes.sante.fr, 27 April 2012 (version dated 6 November 2013 on Internet Archive).

5. Global Burden of disease [database].washington, DC: institute of Health. Metrics, 2019 IHME

6. United States Department of Health and Human Services. The Health Consequences of Smoking: Cancer. A Report of the Surgeon General. United States Department of Health and Human Services, Public Health Service, Office on Smoking and Health. DHHS Publication no (PHS) 82-50179, 1982.

7. Smoking (active or passive) in relation to fertility, medically assisted reproduction and pregnancy J. Berthiller*, A.-J. Sasco/ J Gynecol Obstet Biol Reprod 2005; 34: 3S47-3S54.

8. Braillon A. Violence during pregnancy. What about smoking? Acta Obstet Gynecol Scand 2009: 17.

9. Consequences of tobacco, cocaine and cannabis consumption during pregnancy on the pregnancy itself, on the newborn and on child development : A review S. Lamy , X. Laqueille, F. Thibaut 2015

10. United States. Public Health Service. Office of the Surgeon General. Rockville, MD: US Dept of Health and Human Services, Public Health Service, Office of the Surgeon General; 2001. Women and Smoking: A Report of the Surgeon General.

11. Cornelius MD. Adolescent pregnancy and the complications of prenatal

substance use. Physical and Occupational Therapy in Pediatrics 1996;16(1-2):111-23.

12. Euro-peristat. European Perinatal Health Report 2008. (online) available at http://www.europeristat.com/bm.doc/european-perinatalhealth-report.pdf consulted on 26 April 2023

13. World Health Organization. (2021). WHO global report on trends in prevalence of tobacco use 2000-2025 (4th ed). World Health Organization (online) available at https://www.who.int/publications/i/item/9789240039322 accessed on 04 June 2023

14. GSTHR. (2022). Smoking, vaping, HTP, NRT and snus in Lesotho. Global State of Tobacco Harm Reduction. (online) available at https://gsthr.org/countries/profile/lso/1/ consulted on 15 November 2023

15. Ministry of Planning and Monitoring the Implementation of the Modernity Revolution, Ministry of Public Health and ICF International. Demographic and health survey in the Democratic Republic of Congo 2013-2014. 2014. https://dhsprogram.com/methodology/survey/survey-display-421.cfm

16. C. FARBIER. Histoire du tabac et ses persécutions ; Librairie moderne 19, Boulevard de sebastopol, Rive gauche Gustave Havard, Éditeur 1861/Paris.

17. Rose-Marie Bouboutou, "Cinq choses à savoir sur le tabac en Afrique" (online) available at https://www.bbc.com/afrique/48472738 consulted on 09 January 2023

18. P. AArvers,G. Matherna , Dautzenberg. Les anciens et nouveaux produits du tabac/Old and new tobacco products. Journal of clinical pulmonology 2018

19. Pechacek TF, Folsom AR, de Gaudermaris R, Jacobs Jr DR, et al. Smoke exposure in pipe and cigar smokers serum thiocyanate measures. JAMA 1985 ;254 :3330 - 2.

20. French Monitoring Centre for Drugs and Drug Addiction. Baromètre santé tabac. Saint Maurice: Santé Publique France; 2017 (online) available at http://www.ofdt.fr/pdf/586 consulted on 20 April 2023

21. Koszowski B, Rosenberry ZR, Viray LC, Potts JL, Pickworth WB. Make your own cigarettes: toxicant exposure, smoking topography, and subjective effects. Cancer Epidemiol Biomarkers Prev 2014 ; 23 :1793 - 803

22. Darrall KG, Figgins JA. Roll-your-own smoke yields: theoretical and practical aspects. Tob Control 1998 ;7 : 168 - 75.

23. Appel BR, Guirguis G, Kim IS, Garbin O, Fracchia M, Flessel CP, et al. Benzene, benzo(a)pyrene, and lead in smoke from tobacco products other than cigarettes. Am J Public Health 1990; 80: 560 - 4.

24. Shahab L, West R, McNeill A. A comparison of exposure to carcinogens among roll-your-own and factory-made cigarette smokers. Addict Biol 2009; 14:315 - 20

25. Tabac Info Service. Passive smoking (online) available at http://www.tabac-info-service.fr consulted on 17 May 2023

26. Dautzenberg B. Report of the DGS working group. Passive smoking. 2001. (online) available at http://www.ladocumentationfrancaise.fr/var/storage/rapportspublics/014000432.pdf

27. Hukkanen, J., Pleyton, J. and Benowitz, N.L. (2005). Metabolism and disposition kinetics of nicotine. Pharmacological Reviews, 57(1), 79-115

28. Wall, M.A., Johnson, J., Jacon, P. and Benowitz, N.L. (1988). Cotinine in the serum, saliva, and urine of nonsmokers, passive smokers, and active smokers. American Journal of Public Health, 78,699-701.

29. Murphy, S.E., Link, C.A., Jensen, J., Le, C., Puumala, S.S., Hecht, S.S., Carmella, S.G., Losey, L. and Hatsukami, D.K. (2004). A comparison of urinary biomarkers of tobacco and carcinogen exposure in smokers. Cancer Epidemiology, Biomarkers and Prevention, 13(10), 1617-23.

30. Brown, K., von Weymarn, L. and Murphy, S. (2005). Identification of N-(hydroxymethyl) norcotinine as a major product of cytochrome P450 2A6, but not cytochrome P450 2A13-catalyzed cotinine metabolism. Chemical Research

in Toxicology, 18(12), 1792-98.

31. Etzel, R.A. (1990). A review of the use of saliva cotinine as a marker of tobacco smoke exposure. Preventive Medicine, 19(2), 190-7.

32. Florek, E., Piekoszewski, W. and Wrzosek, J. (2003). Relationship between the level and time of exposure to tobacco smoke and urine nicotine and cotinine concentration. Polish Journal of Pharmacology, 55, 97-102.

33. Nakajima, M., Yamamoto, T., Nunoya, K., Yokoi, T., Nagashima, K., Inoue, K., Funae, Y., Shimada, N., Kamataki, T. and Kuroiwa, Y. (1996). Role of human cytochrome P4502A6 in C-oxidation of nicotine. Drug Metabolism and Disposition. 24(11), 1212-17.

34. Wong, S.L., Shields, M., Leatherdale, S., Malaison, E., & Hammond, D. (2012). Assessing the validity self-reported smoking status. Health Reports, Statistics Canada, 23(1), 1-8.

35. Consensus Conference on Pregnancy and Tobacco 7 and 8 October 2004 Lille (Grand Palais) TEXT OF RECOMMENDATIONS (on line) available at http://www.has-santé.fr consulted on 20 May 2023

36. Greaves, L., Cormier, R., Devries, K., Bottorff, J., Johnson, J., Kirkland, S., Aboussafy, D. Smoking Cessation and Pregnancy. A review of smoking cessation best practices for girls and women during pregnancy and the postpartum period Vancouver British Columbia Centre of Excellence for Women's Health. 2003

37. Cornelius MD Day NL. Developmental consequences of prenatal tobacco exposure. Curr Opin Neurol. 2009 ; 22(2) :121 - 5.

38. Yang C Shooshtari S Oubliez EL Clara I Cheung K. Smoking during pregnancy: findings from the 2009-2010 Canadian Community Health Survey. PloS One. 2014 ; 9(1) : E84640.

39. Tong, VT, Dietz, PM Morrow, B et al. Trends in smoking before, during, and after pregnancy: Pregnancy Risk Assessment Surveillance System, United States, 40 sites, 2000-2010. 2013. (online) available at http://www.cdc.gov/mmwr/preview/mmwrhtml/ss6206a1 accessed on 30 April

2023

40. Chazeron I de, Llorca P-M, Ughetto S, Coudore F, Boussiron D, Perriot J, et al. Occult maternal exposure to environmental tobacco smoke exposure. Tob Control. 2007 Feb 1;16(1):64 -5

41. Aurrekoetxea JJ, Murcia M, Rebagliato M, Fernández-Somoano A, Castilla AM, Guxens M, López MJ, Lertxundi A, Espada M, Tardón A, Ballester F, Santa-Marina L. Factors associated with exposure to second-hand smoke in non-smoking pregnant women in Spain: self-reported exposure and urinary cotinine levels. Sci Total Environ. 2014 Feb 1;470-1.

42. Maïté BRU. Screening and obstetric consequences of carbon monoxide poisoning in the delivery room/ université Claude BERNARD LYON I /UFR de Médecine maieutique LYON sud Charles Mérieux /promotion 2010-2014 page 31

43. Conchita GOMEZ-DELCROIX. Tobacco smoke and the impact of cadmium and carbon monoxide on foeto-placental development/ University of Limoges ED 615 - Biological Sciences and Health (SBS) IPPRIT-UMR INSERM - CHU 1248/ 22 September 2022

44. Agnès Dumas. TOBACCO, PREGNANCY AND BREASTFEEDING: AN EXHIBITION, KNOWLEDGE AND PERCEPTIONS OF RISKS/ Centre de recherche en épidémiologie et santé des populations (CESP), Inserm U1018, Villejuif, France 2 Cermes3, UMR 8/ 2014.

45. S. Lamy, X. Laqueille, F. Thibaut Consequences of tobacco, cocaine and cannabis consumption during pregnancy on the pregnancy itself, on the newborn and on child development. DOI: 10.1016/j.encep.2014.08.012. EPUB 2014 October 28

46. GRANGE et al. Rapport d'experts et recommandations CNGOF-SFT sur la prise en charge du tabagisme en cours de grossesse -texte court ; Gynécologie Obstétrique Fertilité & Sénologie ; 2020, (7) : 539-45.

47. Brian A. Primack, MD, Mary V, Carroll RN, Patricia M, Weiss, MLISc Alan

L. et al. Systematic Review and Meta-Analysis of Inhaled Toxicants from Waterpipe and Cigarette Smoking/Public Health Reports / January-February 2016 / Volume 131

48. V. Dochez, C. Diguisto. Epidemiology and risk factors of tobacco consumption during pregnancy (excluding coaddictions) ; Gynécologie Obstétrique Fertilité & Sénologie. 2020 (48) : 546-50.

APPENDIX

I. IDENTIFICATION OF THE RESPONDENT

N°	Variable	Modality	Code
Q1	Name postname and first name	....	
Q2	Telephone	....	
Q3	Recruitment date	....	
Q4	Address	....	
Q5	Province origin		
Q6	Health structure		
Q7	Health zone		

II.DEMOGRAPHIC PARAMETERS

N°	Variable	Modality	Code
Q8	Age	... years	
Q9	Gender	1=M 2=F	
Q10	Civil status	1= single 2= married 3= divorced 4= widower	
Q11	Profession	1= unemployed 2= company officer 3= Business executive 4= Military 5=Doctor 6=Lawyer 7=Engineer 8=Housekeeper 9=Other	
Q12	Level of study	1= never attended school 2= primary 3= secondary 4= vocational 5= university 6= Other	
Q13	Religious confession	1= Catholic 2= Protestant 3=Kimbanguist 4=Muslim 5= Revival church 6= Other	

III. History of G.O. and cardiovascular risk factors

N°	Variable	Modality	Code
Q14	Parity		
Q15	Gestité		
Q16	Abortions	1 = Yes 2 = No If yes, spontaneous Or induced If yes, number of abortions: When:.................	
Q17	Caesarean section	1= yes 2= no If so, how many caesarean sections ..	
Q18	Notion of EP	1= yes 2= no If yes, how many EPs:...... When:	
Q19	Age of pregnancy		
Q20	Age of last child		
	Last child weight		
Q21	HTA (years)	1= yes 2= no If yes, duration of HAH......years.........months	
Q22	Current pre-eclampsia	1= yes 2= no	
Q23	Atcds of pre-eclampsia	1 = Yes 2= no If yes, how many ...	
Q24	HRP	1 = Yes 2= no If yes, how many ...	
Q25	Placenta previa	1 = Yes 2= no If yes, how many ...	
Q26	Premature delivery	1 = Yes 2= no If yes, how many ...	
Q27	RPM	1 = Yes 2= no If yes, how many ...	
Q28	Neonatal malformation	1= yes 2= no If yes, which one and how many times	
Q29	IUGR	1 = Yes 2= no If yes, how many times	
Q30	Do you drink alcohol?	1=Yes 2=No If yes, since when? .... If yes, go to Q 42	
Q31	Why drink beer?	....	

IV. Lifestyle

N°	Variable	Modality	Code
Q32	Do you know about tobacco ?	1=Yes 2=No.	
Q33	Do you smoke?	1=Yes 2=No. If yes go to 34-38	
Q34	What type of tobacco		
Q35	How many times a day		
Q36	Quantity per day		
Q37	Since when?		
Q38	Why do you smoke?		
Q39	Do you know the risks of smoking?	1= yes 2= no If so, which ones:........	
Q40	Does your partner smoke?	1= yes 2= no If yes, since when ...... If yes, go to Q 41	
Q41	How much per day		
Q42	Do you know anyone who uses tobacco?	1= yes 2= no If yes, go to Q 43	
Q43	How much per day		
Q44	Can give up smoking?	1=Yes 2= no If yes Definitely? Or during pregnancy?	

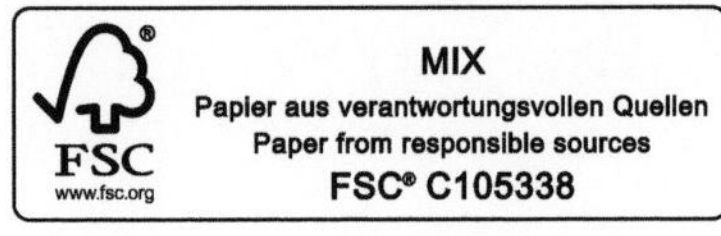

Printed by Books on Demand GmbH, Norderstedt / Germany